# WHY MACROBIOTICS?

## Edward Esko

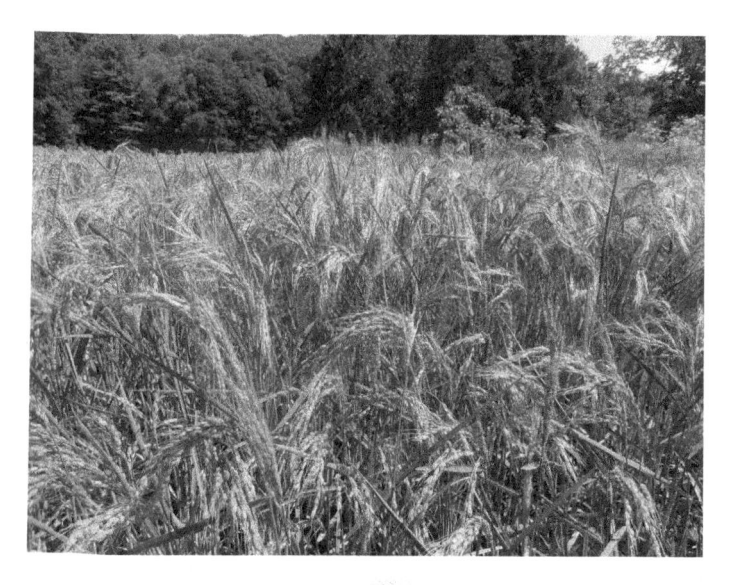

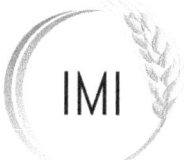

**IMI Press**
InternationalMacrobioticInstitute.com

# WHAT IS MACROBIOTICS?

**Contents**
Introduction     3
Ecological Eating     5
Changing with Our Environment     7
Respecting Human Needs     9
Food as Energy     12
Dietary Diversity     15
Benefits of Macrobiotics     17
About the Author     21

**What Is Macrobiotics?**
Copyright © 2017 Edward Esko
ISBN-13: 978-1981241040
ISBN-10: 1981241043

Published by IMI Press
P.O. Box 2051
Lenox, MA 01240

InternationalMacrobioticInstitute.com

# Introduction

The contents of this small book are taken from a lecture I gave at the Macrobiotic Summer Conference held in Vermont in 1994. The lecture was titled, "Basics and Benefits of Macrobiotics." The lecture was published as a small book and later included in *Contemporary Macrobiotics*, a collection of my essays first published in 2000.

In the lecture I presented the foundational principles of the macrobiotic way of life, including those of ecological eating, eating, selecting and preparing foods in harmony with the environment, respecting human needs and individual requirements, the understanding of the energy of food, and the importance of diversity in the human diet.

The lecture also included an outline of the benefits of living according to these principles, including health and longevity, peace of mind, individual, family, and social peace and stability, spiritual awareness, and ultimately, the freedom to realize and enjoy our fullest potential as a human being.

These principles are as valid today as they were then, and are in fact timeless. They can help serve as a guide to individuals and society as a whole as we navigate the troubled and uncertain waters of the 21st century.

Macrobiotics is founded on the eternal order of change recognized and identified by spiritual leaders and humanist thinkers throughout history. In modern times it was developed and promoted by teachers such as George and Lima Ohsawa, Michio and Aveline Kushi, Herman and Cornelia Aihara, and others. I had the good fortune to know and study personally with these pioneers (with the exception of George Ohsawa who passed in 1966), and owe them all a tremendous debt of gratitude. They pointed the way toward health, peace, and individual freedom amidst the darkness and confusion of modern civilization.

Macrobiotics is a continually evolving search for truth, freedom, knowledge, and justice. By definition, there can be no one fixed, absolute, or static definition since the universe is constantly in motion, and constantly changing. The principles outlined in these pages are merely a guideline or a seed for your evolving practice of this timeless way of life. Please develop your own definition of macrobiotics. My hope is that these principles can guide you toward a bright and healthy future and guide our world toward a future of health and peace for all.

Edward Esko
Pittsfield and Lenox, Mass.
December 2017

# Ecological Eating

One of the most basic principles of macrobiotics is to eat an ecological, environmentally-based diet. That means to rely primarily on foods native to the climate and environment in which we live. Until the modern age, people were more or less dependent on the products of their regional agriculture. Foods that grew in their area formed the basis of their daily diet. It was not until modern technology that it became possible for people to base their diets on foods from regions with far different climates.

Today, it is common for people to consume bananas from South America, sugar from the Caribbean, pineapples from the South Pacific, or kiwi from New Zealand. However, our health depends on our ability to adapt to the changes in our environment. When we eat foods from a climate that is very different from ours, we lose that adaptability. As society moved away from its traditional, ecologically-based diet, there has been a corresponding rise in chronic illness. Therefore, for optimal health, we need to return to a way of eating based on foods produced in our local environment, or at least on foods grown in a climate that is similar to ours.

Foods with more yang, or contracted energy remain viable longer and can come from a greater distance than foods with more yin, or expansive energy. Sea salt and sea vegetables are examples. They are rich in contracted minerals and can come from the oceans around the world, provided these waters are within your hemisphere. Grains, especially with the outer husk attached, remain intact for a long time, even thousands of years, and can come from anywhere in your continent. Beans also travel well and can come from a similarly wide area. However, vegetables and fruits are more yin or expansive; they decompose more rapidly than grains and beans, and unless they are naturally dried or pickled, are best taken from your immediate area.

# Changing with Our Environment

It is also important to adapt our cooking and eating to seasonal changes. The modern way of eating does not do this, as people eat pretty much the same diet throughout the year. High temperatures and bright sunshine produce a stronger charge of upward energy in the environment. Water evaporates more rapidly and plants become lush and expanded. Spring and summer are times of upward, expansive energy. Then toward the end of summer, energy starts to change, moving downward and inward. In colder and darker conditions, such as those of autumn and winter, downward or contracting energy is stronger.

How can we adapt to these changes? During spring and summer, we can make our diet lighter and fresher, meaning that we use less fire in cooking. We do not need as much fire in our cooking because fire is already there in the form of strong sunshine. When it is hot, we do not need warmth from our food. As we move into autumn and winter, with cooler temperatures and stronger downward energy, we make our food hearty and warming by using more fire in cooking.

As the seasons change, we also need to utilize the natural products of our environment. Our gardens are filled with vegetables and other foods during the spring and summer, so we can naturally eat plenty of fresh garden produce during these times. For example, summer is the time when corn is readily available, so it is fine to eat plenty of fresh corn in that season.

From season to season, atmospheric energy alternates as part of the daily cycle. Upward energy is stronger in the morning, while downward energy is stronger in the afternoon and evening. In order to eat in harmony with this cycle, breakfast should be light, not heavy. A breakfast of eggs and bacon is dense and heavy, and goes against the movement of energy. Breakfast grains can be cooked with more water, so that they become lighter and more easily digested. Dinner can include a greater number of side dishes, and we normally eat more in the evening, since at that time, atmospheric energy is more condensed and inward-moving. Lunch can also be quick and light, since at noon, atmospheric energy is very active and expansive. Quick light cooking, such as that in which we reheat leftovers, can be done at that time.

# Respecting Human Needs

Another important principle is to eat according to our distinctive needs as a species. Our teeth reveal the ideal proportion of foods in the human diet. We have thirty-two adult teeth. There are twenty molars and premolars. The word *molar* is a Latin word for *millstone*, or the stones used to crush wheat and other grains into flour. These teeth are not suited for animal food, but for crushing or grinding grains, beans, seeds, and other tough plant fibers. There are also eight front incisors (from the Latin, *to cut*) and these are well-suited for cutting vegetables. We also have four canine teeth. The canines can be used for animal food, not necessarily meat, but foods such as white-meat fish. The ideal proportion of foods as reflected in the teeth is five parts grain and other tough fibrous foods, two parts vegetables, and one part animal food. The ideal ratio between plant and animal food is seven to one.

The modern diet does not reflect this pattern. Rather than whole grains, meat or other types of animal food are the primary foods. Vegetables are often used as garnish to the main course of animal food. Cereal grains are eaten almost as an afterthought, and are eaten in the form of white bread, white rolls, and other highly refined products. Refined bread or rolls are used simply as a vehicle to carry a hot dog, hamburger, or some other type of animal food. Grains are an incidental part of the modern diet.

Today, people are eating the opposite of what they should be eating. That is why so many health problems exist in the modern world. One of the clearest messages I received from the books of George Ohsawa was that plant-based diets are superior to animal-based diets. When Ohsawa presented that idea many years ago, Western doctors and nutritionists laughed. They believed that animal protein was superior to plant protein, and that cultures in which animal protein formed the basis of the diet were more advanced than cultures that relied on grains and other plant foods.

However, that view is changing. The vanguard of modern nutrition now agrees that plant-based diets are better for our health. If we compare the health patterns of people who are eating plant-based diets with those who are eating animal food, the grain- and vegetable-eaters have far lower rates of chronic disease. There is an exception to this of course. If you would like to eat animal food, it would be better for you to move to the Far North, above the Arctic Circle. Then you can eat plenty of animal food. But if you live in Houston, where it is a hundred degrees in the summer, then it is out of order to eat barbecued steak. It does not fulfill our biological needs nor does it make our condition harmonious with our environment.

Macrobiotics also recommends respecting dietary tradition. In the Bible we read, "give us this day our daily bread." Bread is symbolic of grain itself. Wheat, barley, and other grains were considered the staff of life. In the Far East, rice was considered the staple food, the staff of life. Native Americans respected corn as their staff of life. Wherever you look, no matter what your tradition is, if you go back far enough, you find that your ancestors were eating grains as their principal foods. They used local vegetables and beans as secondary foods. They were eating much less animal food than at present.

Nightshade vegetables, especially tomatoes and potatoes, were originally not a part of the diet in Europe. These vegetables were brought to Europe from Peru. The original Italian diet did not include tomato sauce. It was very close to a macrobiotic diet. Originally they did not use much meat; they used more seafood, because Italy is a peninsula. They did not use butter, but used olive oil in cooking. Instead of umeboshi plums, they used pickled olives.

The basis of the diet was whole grain pasta and rice. As people abandoned these traditional eating patterns in favor of the modern diet, their rates of degenerative disease, especially heart disease and cancer, increased dramatically.

# Food as Energy

The practice of macrobiotics is based on the understanding of food as energy. Electrons and protons are not solid particles, but condensed packets of energy. Everything is actually energy, everything is composed of vibration. There is no unchanging or fixed substance in the universe. Therefore, our understanding of food incorporates, but is not limited to, theories of modern nutrition. In modern nutrition, food is viewed as matter. In reality, there is an invisible quality to food (and to life itself) that cannot be measured scientifically. We must perceive that invisible quality directly through our intuition.

In macrobiotics, we employ a very simple tool for understanding the movement of energy. We understand food in terms of yin (expansion) and yang (contraction). All foods are made up of varying degrees of these two basic forces. We use this understanding to see how food affects us in a very dynamic and practical way. By understanding food as energy, we see that it affects not only our physical condition, but our mind, emotions, and even our spirituality. These invisible aspects of life are a function of the quality of energy we manifest.

If we eat a food such as steak, which is very yang or contracted, we are naturally attracted to foods with the opposite quality of energy. So we eat the steak with potatoes, alcohol, or a sugary dessert such as ice cream. All of these foods are extremely yin. In order to balance extremes, we have to add many things that we don't need. We wind up taking in excess fat, excess protein, excess carbohydrate, and excess water. Our body is constantly being challenged.

However, what happens when our main food is more balanced? If you look at a nutritional analysis of whole grains--brown rice, barley, millet, whole wheat--you discover that their ratio of minerals to protein and protein to carbohydrate approximates one to seven. Short grain brown rice comes closest to the one to seven ratio, that, nutritionally speaking, represents the balancing point between expansive and contractive energies on the planet. If you eat whole grains every day, your main foods are balanced in themselves. It is much easier to balance yin and yang in your diet as a whole. Eating whole grains as your primary food makes it much easier to maintain optimal nutritional and energetic balance.

Macrobiotics recommends that our foods be as natural as possible. Today, however, people are using poor quality table salt, treated city water, animal protein instead of plant protein, saturated animal fat instead of vegetable oil, chemically processed rather than organic foods, and plenty of simple sugars instead of complex carbohydrates. It is no wonder that modern people's health is suffering, because the quality of each of these nutritional factors is poor.

The understanding of food as energy can guide us not only in creating an optimal diet, but in the use of simple home remedies for the relief of illness. For example, suppose someone has a kidney stone. What type of energy does that represent, more expansive, yin energy or more condensed, yang energy? A kidney stone is condensed, something like hard, frozen energy. In order to offset that, we need to apply something with the opposite, activating energy. Should we apply heat or cold? We should apply heat. Heat will activate this frozen energy and make it melt and break down. A hot ginger compress can be applied for that purpose.

Fever represents the opposite type of energy. Fever is an example of hot, overactive energy. What would balance that? Something with cool, inert energy. Ice is too cold for this purpose. Ice is so cold that it makes the body contract, so that the excess that is trying to come out through the fever will, instead, be held inside. Something a little milder is needed. Also, our body is part of the animal world, so something from the plant kingdom helps to make balance. A simple macrobiotic remedy for fever is to apply a cabbage leaf or another leafy green directly to the forehead. Another remedy is to take raw tofu, which is cool and inert, mash it, and apply it to the forehead. This application, known as a tofu plaster, draws heat out of the body. It can lower a fever in a matter of minutes. The principle of energy balance can help you manage a variety of minor conditions at home without aspirin or other medications.

# Dietary Diversity

Macrobiotics also teaches that we respect biodiversity, or the tremendous proliferation of life on earth. Many people are concerned with preserving the wealth of species on our planet because biodiversity is now being threatened by civilization. Many species, including those in tropical rain forests, are disappearing. Others are in danger. Scientists have discovered that amphibians such as frogs and salamanders are diminishing, perhaps because of ozone depletion or acid rain. The tiger, the symbol of power and beauty, is vanishing from the wild. However, in nature, biodiversity is the rule, not the exception. To reflect this in our eating, we need to practice what I call *dietary diversity*. There is a wide proliferation of life on earth, a wide range of species, and to translate that into our day to day eating, we need plenty of variety in our selection of foods, and also in our cooking methods. Macrobiotic eating is not narrow or strict. Through macrobiotics, we discover a wide range of healthful new foods.

We also need to respect the endless diversity of individual needs. Although we share certain fundamental things in common, each of us is different. If we are active, we should eat a certain way for physical activity. If we are sitting behind a desk, our diet should be somewhat different. Men and women also need to eat differently. Between men and women, who can eat more animal food? Men. Who can eat more raw salad and sweets? Women. Children and adults also need to eat differently. Babies are already yang--small and contracted--so their diets need to be more yin--soft and sweet-tasting, with little or no salt. If you have eaten plenty of animal food in the past, in order to restore balance, you need to base your diet on plant foods. Or if you have a health problem caused by your past way of eating, you can emphasize certain foods in order to offset that.

# Benefits of Macrobiotics

Now, what are the benefits of macrobiotic living? Eating this way can help us maintain optimal health and achieve longevity. People such as the Hunza in Kashmir, known for their good health and longevity, eat grains and vegetables as their main food. They were eating more or less a macrobiotic diet adapted to their mountainous terrain and climate. The first benefit of macrobiotic eating is physical health and longevity.

A second benefit is peace of mind. That peace of mind comes from the awareness that we are living and eating in harmony with the universe. We are living in harmony with the movement of energy. That is the source of inner peace. Our mind and emotions are very much conditioned by what we eat. If you feed your child plenty of sugar, what kind of mind or emotions result? Children become hyperactive or cry a lot, and become overly emotional. If we eat plenty of meat, what kind of mind and emotions are produced? We become aggressive or in the extreme, even violent. What happens when we eat plenty of nightshade vegetables such as tomatoes or potatoes? We become depressed. Incidentally, these vegetables have recently been found to contain nicotine. Nicotine is an addictive substance, and that may explain why many people find it difficult to stop eating these vegetables.

As your mind and emotions become more stable and peaceful, you naturally develop a sense of family and community. Modern values--such as competition, dog eat dog, survival of the fittest, etc.-- have all arisen from a carnivorous diet. Grain-eating people develop a completely opposite view. Instead of seeing scarcity on the earth, we realize that we live in a universe of abundance. Rather than fighting over resources, the issue becomes how to share the tremendous natural wealth on our planet. Meat-eating tends to produce isolation, something like the lone hunter or lone wolf, rather than a sense of community. Hunters such as lions and hyenas are constantly fighting with each other. Grain-eaters develop a completely opposite way of thinking based on cooperation.

Meat-eating also leads to a more nomadic lifestyle, following the herd, and we tend to become unsettled, rather than stable or settled down. Grain-eating agricultural life is more stable, more settled. Which way of life encourages more stable family life? When the men are off hunting all season, or if the entire village has to constantly be on the move, it is difficult to maintain stability. Macrobiotic living strengthens our community and family life. People naturally desire to help and support each other. Through macrobiotics, you become friends with everyone. As we continue to eat this way, our concept of family expands to include all of humanity. We reconnect with our human family on planet earth.

Macrobiotic living can also help us gain spiritual understanding. Do you think it is easy to meditate if we eat hamburgers, or if our mind is very angry or upset, or if we are always stressed out? Or if we are eating sugar or drinking Coke all the time, so that our mind is often hyperactive and scattered, can we really stabilize and center our energy? These conditions make if very difficult to enter into deep, tranquil, and peaceful meditation. In order to allow spiritual energy to smoothly channel through us, and to use that energy, macrobiotic eating--grains and vegetables--is ideal.

We should not forget that all great spiritual traditions included some form of dietary discipline. In the Orient, the cooking in Buddhist and Taoist monasteries was called *shojin ryiori*, or "cooking for spiritual development." These traditions were based on the understanding that food accelerates our spiritual consciousness. By selecting the proper food, we develop our spiritual quality. In these traditions, do you think animal food was a part of their diets? No. They were completely vegetarian. However, in traditional times, vegetarian eating, especially in cooler climates, meant eating cooked brown rice, daikon and other vegetables, tofu and bean products, etc., rather than a lot of raw fruit or salad.

Finally, as we achieve good health, peace of mind, a sense of family and community, and spiritual understanding, we gain the ability to play and have a big dream or adventure in this life. Macrobiotics is based on change or transmutation. In other words, we try to gain the ability to change things into their opposite according to our free will.

So if we are experiencing difficulty, using macrobiotic understanding, we try to change that into pleasure or enjoyment. Or if we are experiencing sickness, we self-transform that into health. Or if the world is in danger of war, as our adventure, as our play, as our challenge, we transform that into peace. You can even gain the ability to transmute or transform any type of food into your health and vitality. In other words, you embrace your antagonist and turn it into your friend. As George Ohsawa said, ultimately there are no restrictions. The realization of total freedom, or the freedom to play endlessly in this infinite universe, is the ultimate benefit of macrobiotic living.

# About the Author

**Edward Esko** is one of the world's leading teachers and counselors on the macrobiotic way of life. He studied with Michio Kushi and served as Executive Director of the East West Foundation in Boston and Director of Education and Dean of Faculty at the Kushi Institute of the Berkshires. Edward founded the International Macrobiotic Institute (IMI) in 2016 to make quality macrobiotic education and guidance available around the world. He is the founder and creator of the Macrobiotic Online Course and the Nine Star Ki Online Course, and is a member of the Board of Planetary Health, Inc., the non-profit sponsor of the annual Macrobiotic Summer Conference.

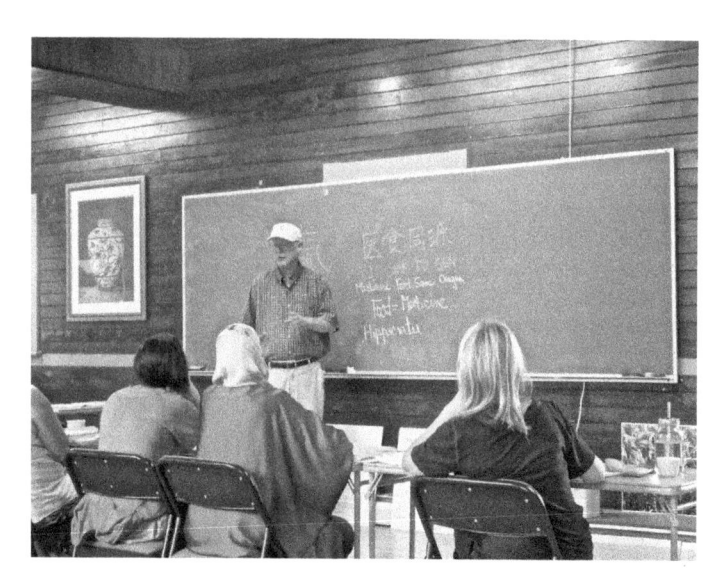

# EDWARD ESKO BOOKS ON AMAZON

*Yin Yang Primer*
*Contemporary Macrobiotics*
*Rice Field Essays*
*Dandelion Essays*
*Ki: The Energy of Life*
*Opening Your Third Eye*
*The Next Twenty Years*
*Ki Balance Massage*
*Food For Peace*
*Macrobiotics (Companion Guide to the Macrobiotic Online Course)*
*Nine Star Ki (Companion Guide to the Nine Star Ki Online Course)*

With Wendy Esko
*Macrobiotic Cooking for Everyone*

With Michio Kushi
*Natural Healing through Macrobiotics*
*Other Dimensions*
*Nine Star Ki*
*The Macrobiotic Approach to Cancer*
*Forgotten Worlds*
*Holistic Health through Macrobiotics*
*Healing Harvest*
*Spiritual Journey*
*The Philosopher's Stone*
*Raising Healthy Kids*
*Basic Shiatsu*
*Dream Diagnosis*

With Alex Jack
*Cool Fusion*
*Corking the Nuclear Genie*
*The Rice Revolution*

Edited by Edward Esko
*Cancer and Heart Disease*
*Crime and Diet*
*Doctors Look at Macrobiotics*
*The Teachings of Michio Kushi*
*Remembering Michio*

# Interested in Using Food as Medicine? Learn From a Master Teacher

Food fuels our body and contains energy that is derived from the sun and our universe. Getting that energy into our body at an optimal level requires an understanding of the Five Transformations and eating seasonally. We adapt our clothing (winter coats, bathing suits), activities (sledding, swimming) and home environment (air conditioning or heat) to the seasons, but why not our food? Our grocery stores carry in-season as well as out-of-season produce. We're used to getting what we want, not waiting to enjoy it when it's at its peak flavor and energy. But what if we eat seasonally, what if we adjust our cooking techniques, what if we choose specific foods to strengthen certain organs? What happens is we realign ourselves to the universe, draw the benefits of its energy and enjoy renewed health.

I've been studying macrobiotics and holistic health with teachers from around the world for almost ten years. I am currently taking a course that has shifted my thinking and has simplified the once confusing concept of food as energy and as medicine to heal. I can't say enough about our teacher, Edward Esko, the Founder of the International Macrobiotic Institute (IMI) and former director of education at the Kushi Institute. Ed has deep knowledge of food energetics and a genuine passion to teach others. The IMI 12 week course combines video, audio, print and live interaction via Skype. I highly recommend this class to everyone interested in deepening their understanding of how to literally use food as medicine. Classes are forming now. For more information visit the International Macrobiotic Institute website. —**Amy Hopeman, Founder, Health Goods Market**

# THE MACROBIOTIC ONLINE COURSE

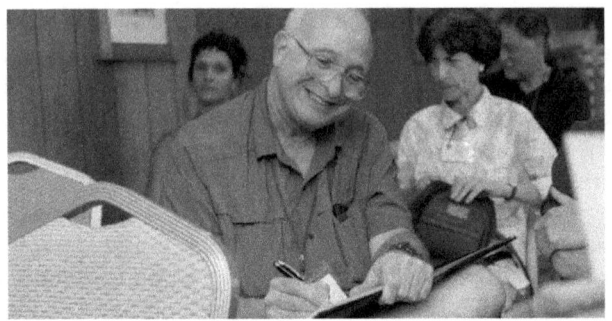

Photo: Nancy Adler

*An online certificate course in macrobiotic teaching, counseling, and guidance*

*"I highly recommend this class to everyone interested in deepening their understanding of how to use food as medicine."*—**Amy Hopeman, MS, MPH, Founder of HealthGoods Market**

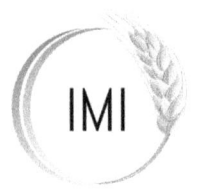

**International Macrobiotic Institute**
Massachusetts * New York * Dubai UAE

InternationalMacrobioticInstitute.com